ALL MY GASTROPARESIS SHIT

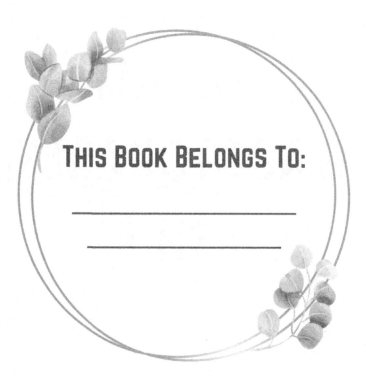

THIS BOOK BELONGS TO:

_____

_____

Date _____

SLEEP QUALITY
ENERGY LEVEL
ACTIVITY LEVEL

LOW   MED   HIGH

MY MOOD

- Relaxed
- Happy
- Inspired
- Angry
- Tired
- Stressed
- _____

TODAY'S GOALS

- _____
- _____
- _____

MEDICATIONS

- _____
- _____
- _____

CURRENT WEIGHT

SUPPLEMENTS

- _____
- _____
- _____

WATER INTAKE

NOTES

_____
_____
_____
_____
_____
_____

FOOD LOG

TIME	FOOD	AMOUNT	CALORIES

TRIGGER TRACKER

IMMEDIATELY AFTER	AFTER 1 HOUR	AFTER 3 HOUR

Date _____

	LOW	MED	HIGH
SLEEP QUALITY	○	○	○
ENERGY LEVEL	○	○	○
ACTIVITY LEVEL	○	○	○

MY MOOD

- ○ Relaxed
- ○ Happy
- ○ Inspired
- ○ Angry
- ○ Tired
- ○ Stressed
- ○ _____

TODAY'S GOALS

- ○ _____
- ○ _____
- ○ _____

MEDICATIONS

- ○ _____
- ○ _____
- ○ _____

SUPPLEMENTS

- ○ _____
- ○ _____
- ○ _____

CURRENT WEIGHT

WATER INTAKE

💧 💧 💧 💧 💧
💧 💧 💧 💧 💧
💧 💧 💧 💧 💧

NOTES

_____
_____
_____
_____
_____
_____

FOOD LOG

TIME	FOOD	AMOUNT	CALORIES

TRIGGER TRACKER

IMMEDIATELY AFTER	AFTER 1 HOUR	AFTER 3 HOUR

Date _____

MY MOOD

SLEEP QUALITY   LOW   MED   HIGH

ENERGY LEVEL

ACTIVITY LEVEL

- Relaxed
- Happy
- Inspired
- Angry
- Tired
- Stressed
- _____

TODAY'S GOALS

- _____
- _____
- _____

MEDICATIONS

- _____
- _____
- _____

CURRENT WEIGHT

SUPPLEMENTS

- _____
- _____
- _____

WATER INTAKE

NOTES

_____
_____
_____
_____
_____
_____

FOOD LOG

TIME	FOOD	AMOUNT	CALORIES

TRIGGER TRACKER

IMMEDIATELY AFTER	AFTER 1 HOUR	AFTER 3 HOUR

Date _____

MY MOOD

- Relaxed
- Happy
- Inspired
- Angry
- Tired
- Stressed
- _____

	LOW	MED	HIGH
SLEEP QUALITY	●	●	●
ENERGY LEVEL	●	●	●
ACTIVITY LEVEL	●	●	●

TODAY'S GOALS

- _____
- _____
- _____

MEDICATIONS

- _____
- _____
- _____

SUPPLEMENTS

- _____
- _____
- _____

CURRENT WEIGHT

WATER INTAKE

NOTES

_____
_____
_____
_____
_____
_____

FOOD LOG

TIME	FOOD	AMOUNT	CALORIES

TRIGGER TRACKER

IMMEDIATELY AFTER	AFTER 1 HOUR	AFTER 3 HOUR

Date _____

MY MOOD

SLEEP QUALITY	LOW	MED	HIGH
ENERGY LEVEL			
ACTIVITY LEVEL			

- Relaxed
- Happy
- Inspired
- Angry
- Tired
- Stressed
- _____

TODAY'S GOALS

- _____
- _____
- _____

MEDICATIONS

- _____
- _____
- _____

CURRENT WEIGHT

WATER INTAKE

SUPPLEMENTS

- _____
- _____
- _____

NOTES

_____
_____
_____
_____
_____
_____
_____

FOOD LOG

TIME	FOOD	AMOUNT	CALORIES

TRIGGER TRACKER

IMMEDIATELY AFTER	AFTER 1 HOUR	AFTER 3 HOUR

Date _____

	LOW	MED	HIGH
SLEEP QUALITY	●	●	●
ENERGY LEVEL	●	●	●
ACTIVITY LEVEL	●	●	●

MY MOOD

● Relaxed
● Happy
● Inspired
● Angry
● Tired
● Stressed
● _____

TODAY'S GOALS

● _____
● _____
● _____

MEDICATIONS

● _____
● _____
● _____

CURRENT WEIGHT

SUPPLEMENTS

● _____
● _____
● _____

WATER INTAKE

💧 💧 💧 💧 💧
💧 💧 💧 💧 💧
💧 💧 💧 💧 💧

NOTES

_____
_____
_____
_____
_____
_____

FOOD LOG

TIME	FOOD	AMOUNT	CALORIES

TRIGGER TRACKER

IMMEDIATELY AFTER	AFTER 1 HOUR	AFTER 3 HOUR

Date _____

	LOW	MED	HIGH
SLEEP QUALITY	●	●	●
ENERGY LEVEL	●	●	●
ACTIVITY LEVEL	●	●	●

MY MOOD

- ● Relaxed
- ● Happy
- ● Inspired
- ● Angry
- ● Tired
- ● Stressed
- ● _____

TODAY'S GOALS

- ● _____
- ● _____
- ● _____

MEDICATIONS

- ● _____
- ● _____
- ● _____

SUPPLEMENTS

- ● _____
- ● _____
- ● _____

CURRENT WEIGHT

WATER INTAKE

💧 💧 💧 💧 💧
💧 💧 💧 💧 💧
💧 💧 💧 💧 💧

NOTES

_____
_____
_____
_____
_____
_____

FOOD LOG

TIME	FOOD	AMOUNT	CALORIES

TRIGGER TRACKER

IMMEDIATELY AFTER	AFTER 1 HOUR	AFTER 3 HOUR

Date _____

	LOW	MED	HIGH
SLEEP QUALITY	●	●	●
ENERGY LEVEL	●	●	●
ACTIVITY LEVEL	●	●	●

MY MOOD

● Relaxed
● Happy
● Inspired
● Angry
● Tired
● Stressed
● _____

TODAY'S GOALS

● _____
● _____
● _____

MEDICATIONS

● _____
● _____
● _____

SUPPLEMENTS

● _____
● _____
● _____

CURRENT WEIGHT

WATER INTAKE

💧 💧 💧 💧 💧
💧 💧 💧 💧 💧
💧 💧 💧 💧 💧

NOTES

_____
_____
_____
_____
_____
_____

FOOD LOG

TIME	FOOD	AMOUNT	CALORIES

TRIGGER TRACKER

IMMEDIATELY AFTER	AFTER 1 HOUR	AFTER 3 HOUR

Date _____

	LOW	MED	HIGH
SLEEP QUALITY	○	○	○
ENERGY LEVEL	○	○	○
ACTIVITY LEVEL	○	○	○

MY MOOD

- Relaxed
- Happy
- Inspired
- Angry
- Tired
- Stressed
- _____

TODAY'S GOALS

- _____
- _____
- _____

MEDICATIONS

- _____
- _____
- _____

SUPPLEMENTS

- _____
- _____
- _____

CURRENT WEIGHT

WATER INTAKE

NOTES

_____
_____
_____
_____
_____
_____

FOOD LOG

TIME	FOOD	AMOUNT	CALORIES

TRIGGER TRACKER

IMMEDIATELY AFTER	AFTER 1 HOUR	AFTER 3 HOUR

Date _____

SLEEP QUALITY / ENERGY LEVEL / ACTIVITY LEVEL

	LOW	MED	HIGH
SLEEP QUALITY	⬤	⬤	⬤
ENERGY LEVEL	⬤	⬤	⬤
ACTIVITY LEVEL	⬤	⬤	⬤

MY MOOD

- ⬤ Relaxed
- ⬤ Happy
- ⬤ Inspired
- ⬤ Angry
- ⬤ Tired
- ⬤ Stressed
- ⬤ _____

TODAY'S GOALS

- ⬤ _____
- ⬤ _____
- ⬤ _____

MEDICATIONS

- ⬤ _____
- ⬤ _____
- ⬤ _____

CURRENT WEIGHT

WATER INTAKE

SUPPLEMENTS

- ⬤ _____
- ⬤ _____
- ⬤ _____

NOTES

_____
_____
_____
_____
_____
_____
_____

FOOD LOG

TIME	FOOD	AMOUNT	CALORIES

TRIGGER TRACKER

IMMEDIATELY AFTER	AFTER 1 HOUR	AFTER 3 HOUR

Date _____

MY MOOD

SLEEP QUALITY	LOW MED HIGH	● ● ●
ENERGY LEVEL		● ● ●
ACTIVITY LEVEL		● ● ●

- ● Relaxed
- ● Happy
- ● Inspired
- ● Angry
- ● Tired
- ● Stressed
- ● _____

TODAY'S GOALS

- ● _____
- ● _____
- ● _____

MEDICATIONS

- ● _____
- ● _____
- ● _____

CURRENT WEIGHT

WATER INTAKE

SUPPLEMENTS

- ● _____
- ● _____
- ● _____

NOTES

_____
_____
_____
_____
_____
_____

FOOD LOG

TIME	FOOD	AMOUNT	CALORIES

TRIGGER TRACKER

IMMEDIATELY AFTER	AFTER 1 HOUR	AFTER 3 HOUR

Date _____

	LOW	MED	HIGH
SLEEP QUALITY	○	○	●
ENERGY LEVEL	○	○	●
ACTIVITY LEVEL	○	○	●

MY MOOD

- ● Relaxed
- ● Happy
- ● Inspired
- ● Angry
- ● Tired
- ● Stressed
- ● _____

TODAY'S GOALS

- ● _____
- ● _____
- ● _____

MEDICATIONS

- ● _____
- ● _____
- ● _____

SUPPLEMENTS

- ● _____
- ● _____
- ● _____

CURRENT WEIGHT

WATER INTAKE

💧 💧 💧 💧 💧
💧 💧 💧 💧 💧
💧 💧 💧 💧 💧

NOTES

_____
_____
_____
_____
_____
_____

FOOD LOG

TIME	FOOD	AMOUNT	CALORIES

TRIGGER TRACKER

IMMEDIATELY AFTER	AFTER 1 HOUR	AFTER 3 HOUR

Date _____

MY MOOD

	LOW	MED	HIGH
SLEEP QUALITY	●	●	●
ENERGY LEVEL	●	●	●
ACTIVITY LEVEL	●	●	●

● Relaxed

● Happy

● Inspired

● Angry

● Tired

● Stressed

● _____

TODAY'S GOALS

● _____

● _____

● _____

MEDICATIONS

● _____

● _____

● _____

CURRENT WEIGHT

WATER INTAKE

SUPPLEMENTS

● _____

● _____

● _____

NOTES

_____
_____
_____
_____
_____
_____

FOOD LOG

TIME	FOOD	AMOUNT	CALORIES

TRIGGER TRACKER

IMMEDIATELY AFTER	AFTER 1 HOUR	AFTER 3 HOUR

Date _____

MY MOOD

		LOW	MED	HIGH
SLEEP QUALITY		●	●	●
ENERGY LEVEL		●	●	●
ACTIVITY LEVEL		●	●	●

● Relaxed

● Happy

● Inspired

● Angry

● Tired

● Stressed

● _____

TODAY'S GOALS

● _____
● _____
● _____

MEDICATIONS

● _____
● _____
● _____

CURRENT WEIGHT

SUPPLEMENTS

● _____
● _____
● _____

WATER INTAKE

NOTES

_____
_____
_____
_____
_____
_____

FOOD LOG

TIME	FOOD	AMOUNT	CALORIES

TRIGGER TRACKER

IMMEDIATELY AFTER	AFTER 1 HOUR	AFTER 3 HOUR

Date _____

MY MOOD

- Relaxed
- Happy
- Inspired
- Angry
- Tired
- Stressed
- _____

	LOW	MED	HIGH
SLEEP QUALITY	●	●	●
ENERGY LEVEL	●	●	●
ACTIVITY LEVEL	●	●	●

TODAY'S GOALS

- _____
- _____
- _____

MEDICATIONS

- _____
- _____
- _____

CURRENT WEIGHT

SUPPLEMENTS

- _____
- _____
- _____

WATER INTAKE

💧 💧 💧 💧 💧
💧 💧 💧 💧 💧
💧 💧 💧 💧 💧

NOTES

_____
_____
_____
_____
_____
_____

FOOD LOG

TIME	FOOD	AMOUNT	CALORIES

TRIGGER TRACKER

IMMEDIATELY AFTER	AFTER 1 HOUR	AFTER 3 HOUR

Date _____

MY MOOD

SLEEP QUALITY LOW MED HIGH
ENERGY LEVEL
ACTIVITY LEVEL

- Relaxed
- Happy
- Inspired
- Angry
- Tired
- Stressed
- _____

TODAY'S GOALS

- _____
- _____
- _____

MEDICATIONS

- _____
- _____
- _____

CURRENT WEIGHT

WATER INTAKE

SUPPLEMENTS

- _____
- _____
- _____

NOTES

_____
_____
_____
_____
_____
_____

FOOD LOG

TIME	FOOD	AMOUNT	CALORIES

TRIGGER TRACKER

IMMEDIATELY AFTER	AFTER 1 HOUR	AFTER 3 HOUR

Date _____

	LOW	MED	HIGH
SLEEP QUALITY	⬤	⬤	⬤
ENERGY LEVEL	⬤	⬤	⬤
ACTIVITY LEVEL	⬤	⬤	⬤

MY MOOD

⬤ Relaxed
⬤ Happy
⬤ Inspired
⬤ Angry
⬤ Tired
⬤ Stressed
⬤ _____

TODAY'S GOALS

- _____
- _____
- _____

MEDICATIONS

- _____
- _____
- _____

CURRENT WEIGHT

SUPPLEMENTS

- _____
- _____
- _____

WATER INTAKE

NOTES

_____
_____
_____
_____
_____
_____

FOOD LOG

TIME	FOOD	AMOUNT	CALORIES

TRIGGER TRACKER

IMMEDIATELY AFTER	AFTER 1 HOUR	AFTER 3 HOUR

Date _____

MY MOOD

- SLEEP QUALITY
- ENERGY LEVEL
- ACTIVITY LEVEL

LOW   MED   HIGH

- Relaxed
- Happy
- Inspired
- Angry
- Tired
- Stressed
- _____

TODAY'S GOALS

- _____
- _____
- _____

MEDICATIONS

- _____
- _____
- _____

CURRENT WEIGHT

WATER INTAKE

SUPPLEMENTS

- _____
- _____
- _____

NOTES

_____
_____
_____
_____
_____
_____

FOOD LOG

TIME	FOOD	AMOUNT	CALORIES

TRIGGER TRACKER

IMMEDIATELY AFTER	AFTER 1 HOUR	AFTER 3 HOUR

Date _____

MY MOOD

SLEEP QUALITY   LOW   MED   HIGH

ENERGY LEVEL

ACTIVITY LEVEL

- Relaxed
- Happy
- Inspired
- Angry
- Tired
- Stressed
- _____

TODAY'S GOALS

- _____
- _____
- _____

MEDICATIONS

- _____
- _____
- _____

CURRENT WEIGHT

WATER INTAKE

SUPPLEMENTS

- _____
- _____
- _____

NOTES

_____
_____
_____
_____
_____
_____

FOOD LOG

TIME	FOOD	AMOUNT	CALORIES

TRIGGER TRACKER

IMMEDIATELY AFTER	AFTER 1 HOUR	AFTER 3 HOUR

Date _____

MY MOOD

- Relaxed
- Happy
- Inspired
- Angry
- Tired
- Stressed
- _____

	LOW	MED	HIGH
SLEEP QUALITY	○	○	○
ENERGY LEVEL	○	○	○
ACTIVITY LEVEL	○	○	○

TODAY'S GOALS

- _____
- _____
- _____

MEDICATIONS

- _____
- _____
- _____

CURRENT WEIGHT

SUPPLEMENTS

- _____
- _____
- _____

WATER INTAKE

NOTES

_____
_____
_____
_____
_____
_____

FOOD LOG

TIME	FOOD	AMOUNT	CALORIES

TRIGGER TRACKER

IMMEDIATELY AFTER	AFTER 1 HOUR	AFTER 3 HOUR

Date _____

	LOW	MED	HIGH
SLEEP QUALITY	●	●	●
ENERGY LEVEL	●	●	●
ACTIVITY LEVEL	●	●	●

MY MOOD

● Relaxed

● Happy

● Inspired

● Angry

● Tired

● Stressed

● _____

TODAY'S GOALS

● _____
● _____
● _____

MEDICATIONS

● _____
● _____
● _____

CURRENT WEIGHT

WATER INTAKE

SUPPLEMENTS

● _____
● _____
● _____

NOTES

_____
_____
_____
_____
_____
_____

FOOD LOG

TIME	FOOD	AMOUNT	CALORIES

TRIGGER TRACKER

IMMEDIATELY AFTER	AFTER 1 HOUR	AFTER 3 HOUR

Date _____

MY MOOD

SLEEP QUALITY   LOW MED HIGH

	LOW	MED	HIGH
SLEEP QUALITY	●	●	●
ENERGY LEVEL	●	●	●
ACTIVITY LEVEL	●	●	●

- ● Relaxed
- ● Happy
- ● Inspired
- ● Angry
- ● Tired
- ● Stressed
- ● _____

TODAY'S GOALS

- ● _____
- ● _____
- ● _____

MEDICATIONS

- ● _____
- ● _____
- ● _____

CURRENT WEIGHT

WATER INTAKE

SUPPLEMENTS

- ● _____
- ● _____
- ● _____

NOTES

_____
_____
_____
_____
_____
_____

FOOD LOG

TIME	FOOD	AMOUNT	CALORIES

TRIGGER TRACKER

IMMEDIATELY AFTER	AFTER 1 HOUR	AFTER 3 HOUR

Date _____

MY MOOD

- Relaxed
- Happy
- Inspired
- Angry
- Tired
- Stressed
- _____

	LOW	MED	HIGH
SLEEP QUALITY	○	○	○
ENERGY LEVEL	○	○	○
ACTIVITY LEVEL	○	○	○

TODAY'S GOALS

- _____
- _____
- _____

MEDICATIONS

- _____
- _____
- _____

CURRENT WEIGHT

SUPPLEMENTS

- _____
- _____
- _____

WATER INTAKE

NOTES

_____
_____
_____
_____
_____
_____

FOOD LOG

TIME	FOOD	AMOUNT	CALORIES

TRIGGER TRACKER

IMMEDIATELY AFTER	AFTER 1 HOUR	AFTER 3 HOUR

Date _____

MY MOOD

SLEEP QUALITY | LOW MED HIGH
ENERGY LEVEL
ACTIVITY LEVEL

- Relaxed
- Happy
- Inspired
- Angry
- Tired
- Stressed
- _____

TODAY'S GOALS

- _____
- _____
- _____

MEDICATIONS

- _____
- _____
- _____

SUPPLEMENTS

- _____
- _____
- _____

CURRENT WEIGHT

WATER INTAKE

NOTES

_____
_____
_____
_____
_____
_____

FOOD LOG

TIME	FOOD	AMOUNT	CALORIES

TRIGGER TRACKER

IMMEDIATELY AFTER	AFTER 1 HOUR	AFTER 3 HOUR

Date _____

	LOW	MED	HIGH
SLEEP QUALITY	●	●	●
ENERGY LEVEL	●	●	●
ACTIVITY LEVEL	●	●	●

MY MOOD

● Relaxed
● Happy
● Inspired
● Angry
● Tired
● Stressed
● _____

TODAY'S GOALS

● _____
● _____
● _____

MEDICATIONS

● _____
● _____
● _____

CURRENT WEIGHT

WATER INTAKE

SUPPLEMENTS

● _____
● _____
● _____

NOTES

_____
_____
_____
_____
_____
_____

FOOD LOG

TIME	FOOD	AMOUNT	CALORIES

TRIGGER TRACKER

IMMEDIATELY AFTER	AFTER 1 HOUR	AFTER 3 HOUR

Date _____

	LOW	MED	HIGH
SLEEP QUALITY	○	○	○
ENERGY LEVEL	○	○	○
ACTIVITY LEVEL	○	○	○

MY MOOD

- Relaxed
- Happy
- Inspired
- Angry
- Tired
- Stressed
- _____

TODAY'S GOALS

- _____
- _____
- _____

MEDICATIONS

- _____
- _____
- _____

CURRENT WEIGHT

SUPPLEMENTS

- _____
- _____
- _____

WATER INTAKE

NOTES

_____
_____
_____
_____
_____
_____

FOOD LOG

TIME	FOOD	AMOUNT	CALORIES

TRIGGER TRACKER

IMMEDIATELY AFTER	AFTER 1 HOUR	AFTER 3 HOUR

Date _____

	LOW	MED	HIGH
SLEEP QUALITY	○	○	○
ENERGY LEVEL	○	○	○
ACTIVITY LEVEL	○	○	○

MY MOOD

- Relaxed
- Happy
- Inspired
- Angry
- Tired
- Stressed
- _____

TODAY'S GOALS

- _____
- _____
- _____

MEDICATIONS

- _____
- _____
- _____

SUPPLEMENTS

- _____
- _____
- _____

CURRENT WEIGHT

WATER INTAKE

NOTES

_____
_____
_____
_____
_____
_____

FOOD LOG

TIME	FOOD	AMOUNT	CALORIES

TRIGGER TRACKER

IMMEDIATELY AFTER	AFTER 1 HOUR	AFTER 3 HOUR

Date _____

MY MOOD

	LOW	MED	HIGH
SLEEP QUALITY	○	○	●
ENERGY LEVEL	○	●	●
ACTIVITY LEVEL	○	●	●

- Relaxed
- Happy
- Inspired
- Angry
- Tired
- Stressed
- _____

TODAY'S GOALS

- _____
- _____
- _____

MEDICATIONS

- _____
- _____
- _____

CURRENT WEIGHT

WATER INTAKE

SUPPLEMENTS

- _____
- _____
- _____

NOTES

_____
_____
_____
_____
_____
_____

FOOD LOG

TIME	FOOD	AMOUNT	CALORIES

TRIGGER TRACKER

IMMEDIATELY AFTER	AFTER 1 HOUR	AFTER 3 HOUR

Date _____

SLEEP QUALITY   LOW   MED   HIGH

ENERGY LEVEL

ACTIVITY LEVEL

MY MOOD
- Relaxed
- Happy
- Inspired
- Angry
- Tired
- Stressed
- _____

TODAY'S GOALS

- _____
- _____
- _____

MEDICATIONS

- _____
- _____
- _____

CURRENT WEIGHT

SUPPLEMENTS

- _____
- _____
- _____

WATER INTAKE

NOTES

_____
_____
_____
_____
_____
_____

FOOD LOG

TIME	FOOD	AMOUNT	CALORIES

TRIGGER TRACKER

IMMEDIATELY AFTER	AFTER 1 HOUR	AFTER 3 HOUR

Date _____

MY MOOD

	SLEEP QUALITY	LOW	MED	HIGH

SLEEP QUALITY ○ ○ ●
ENERGY LEVEL ○ ○ ●
ACTIVITY LEVEL ○ ○ ●

- Relaxed
- Happy
- Inspired
- Angry
- Tired
- Stressed
- _____

TODAY'S GOALS

- _____
- _____
- _____

MEDICATIONS

- _____
- _____
- _____

SUPPLEMENTS

- _____
- _____
- _____

CURRENT WEIGHT

WATER INTAKE

NOTES

_____
_____
_____
_____
_____
_____

FOOD LOG

TIME	FOOD	AMOUNT	CALORIES

TRIGGER TRACKER

IMMEDIATELY AFTER	AFTER 1 HOUR	AFTER 3 HOUR

Date _____

MY MOOD

SLEEP QUALITY   LOW   MED   HIGH

ENERGY LEVEL

ACTIVITY LEVEL

- Relaxed
- Happy
- Inspired
- Angry
- Tired
- Stressed
- _____

TODAY'S GOALS

- _____
- _____
- _____

MEDICATIONS

- _____
- _____
- _____

CURRENT WEIGHT

WATER INTAKE

SUPPLEMENTS

- _____
- _____
- _____

NOTES

_____
_____
_____
_____
_____
_____

FOOD LOG

TIME	FOOD	AMOUNT	CALORIES

TRIGGER TRACKER

IMMEDIATELY AFTER	AFTER 1 HOUR	AFTER 3 HOUR

Date _____

MY MOOD

- Relaxed
- Happy
- Inspired
- Angry
- Tired
- Stressed
- _____

	LOW	MED	HIGH
SLEEP QUALITY	○	○	○
ENERGY LEVEL	○	○	○
ACTIVITY LEVEL	○	○	○

TODAY'S GOALS

- _____
- _____
- _____

MEDICATIONS

- _____
- _____
- _____

CURRENT WEIGHT

SUPPLEMENTS

- _____
- _____
- _____

WATER INTAKE

NOTES

_____
_____
_____
_____
_____
_____

FOOD LOG

TIME	FOOD	AMOUNT	CALORIES

TRIGGER TRACKER

IMMEDIATELY AFTER	AFTER 1 HOUR	AFTER 3 HOUR

Date _____

SLEEP QUALITY   LOW MED HIGH
ENERGY LEVEL   ○   ○   ○
ACTIVITY LEVEL   ○   ○   ○

MY MOOD

- Relaxed
- Happy
- Inspired
- Angry
- Tired
- Stressed
- _____

TODAY'S GOALS

- _____
- _____
- _____

MEDICATIONS

- _____
- _____
- _____

CURRENT WEIGHT

WATER INTAKE

SUPPLEMENTS

- _____
- _____
- _____

NOTES

_____
_____
_____
_____
_____
_____

FOOD LOG

TIME	FOOD	AMOUNT	CALORIES

TRIGGER TRACKER

IMMEDIATELY AFTER	AFTER 1 HOUR	AFTER 3 HOUR

Date _____

MY MOOD

SLEEP QUALITY
ENERGY LEVEL
ACTIVITY LEVEL

LOW   MED   HIGH

- Relaxed
- Happy
- Inspired
- Angry
- Tired
- Stressed
- _____

TODAY'S GOALS

- _____
- _____
- _____

MEDICATIONS

- _____
- _____
- _____

CURRENT WEIGHT

WATER INTAKE

SUPPLEMENTS

- _____
- _____
- _____

NOTES

_____
_____
_____
_____
_____
_____

FOOD LOG

TIME	FOOD	AMOUNT	CALORIES

TRIGGER TRACKER

IMMEDIATELY AFTER	AFTER 1 HOUR	AFTER 3 HOUR

Date _____

MY MOOD

SLEEP QUALITY	LOW	MED	HIGH
ENERGY LEVEL	○	○	○
ACTIVITY LEVEL	○	○	○

- Relaxed
- Happy
- Inspired
- Angry
- Tired
- Stressed
- _____

TODAY'S GOALS

- _____
- _____
- _____

MEDICATIONS

- _____
- _____
- _____

CURRENT WEIGHT

WATER INTAKE

SUPPLEMENTS

- _____
- _____
- _____

NOTES

_____
_____
_____
_____
_____
_____

FOOD LOG

TIME	FOOD	AMOUNT	CALORIES

TRIGGER TRACKER

IMMEDIATELY AFTER	AFTER 1 HOUR	AFTER 3 HOUR

Date _____

MY MOOD

- Relaxed
- Happy
- Inspired
- Angry
- Tired
- Stressed
- _____

	LOW	MED	HIGH
SLEEP QUALITY	○	○	○
ENERGY LEVEL	○	○	○
ACTIVITY LEVEL	○	○	○

TODAY'S GOALS

- _____
- _____
- _____

MEDICATIONS

- _____
- _____
- _____

CURRENT WEIGHT

SUPPLEMENTS

- _____
- _____
- _____

WATER INTAKE

NOTES

_____
_____
_____
_____
_____
_____

FOOD LOG

TIME	FOOD	AMOUNT	CALORIES

TRIGGER TRACKER

IMMEDIATELY AFTER	AFTER 1 HOUR	AFTER 3 HOUR

Date _____

MY MOOD

SLEEP QUALITY   LOW   MED   HIGH

ENERGY LEVEL

ACTIVITY LEVEL

- Relaxed
- Happy
- Inspired
- Angry
- Tired
- Stressed
- _____

TODAY'S GOALS

- _____
- _____
- _____

MEDICATIONS

- _____
- _____
- _____

SUPPLEMENTS

- _____
- _____
- _____

CURRENT WEIGHT

WATER INTAKE

NOTES

_____
_____
_____
_____
_____
_____

FOOD LOG

TIME	FOOD	AMOUNT	CALORIES

TRIGGER TRACKER

IMMEDIATELY AFTER	AFTER 1 HOUR	AFTER 3 HOUR

Date _____

MY MOOD

SLEEP QUALITY
ENERGY LEVEL
ACTIVITY LEVEL

LOW   MED   HIGH

- Relaxed
- Happy
- Inspired
- Angry
- Tired
- Stressed
- _____

TODAY'S GOALS

- _____
- _____
- _____

MEDICATIONS

- _____
- _____
- _____

CURRENT WEIGHT

SUPPLEMENTS

- _____
- _____
- _____

WATER INTAKE

NOTES

_____
_____
_____
_____
_____
_____

FOOD LOG

TIME	FOOD	AMOUNT	CALORIES

TRIGGER TRACKER

IMMEDIATELY AFTER	AFTER 1 HOUR	AFTER 3 HOUR

Date _____

MY MOOD

SLEEP QUALITY   LOW   MED   HIGH

ENERGY LEVEL

ACTIVITY LEVEL

- Relaxed
- Happy
- Inspired
- Angry
- Tired
- Stressed
- _____

TODAY'S GOALS

- _____
- _____
- _____

MEDICATIONS

- _____
- _____
- _____

CURRENT WEIGHT

SUPPLEMENTS

- _____
- _____
- _____

WATER INTAKE

NOTES

_____
_____
_____
_____
_____
_____

FOOD LOG

TIME	FOOD	AMOUNT	CALORIES

TRIGGER TRACKER

IMMEDIATELY AFTER	AFTER 1 HOUR	AFTER 3 HOUR

Date _____

MY MOOD

- Relaxed
- Happy
- Inspired
- Angry
- Tired
- Stressed
- _____

	LOW	MED	HIGH
SLEEP QUALITY	●	●	●
ENERGY LEVEL	●	●	●
ACTIVITY LEVEL	●	●	●

TODAY'S GOALS

- _____
- _____
- _____

MEDICATIONS

- _____
- _____
- _____

SUPPLEMENTS

- _____
- _____
- _____

CURRENT WEIGHT

WATER INTAKE

NOTES

_____
_____
_____
_____
_____
_____

FOOD LOG

TIME	FOOD	AMOUNT	CALORIES

TRIGGER TRACKER

IMMEDIATELY AFTER	AFTER 1 HOUR	AFTER 3 HOUR

Date _____

MY MOOD

- Relaxed
- Happy
- Inspired
- Angry
- Tired
- Stressed
- _____

	LOW	MED	HIGH
SLEEP QUALITY	○	○	○
ENERGY LEVEL	○	○	○
ACTIVITY LEVEL	○	○	○

TODAY'S GOALS

- _____
- _____
- _____

MEDICATIONS

- _____
- _____
- _____

SUPPLEMENTS

- _____
- _____
- _____

CURRENT WEIGHT

WATER INTAKE

NOTES

_____
_____
_____
_____
_____
_____

FOOD LOG

TIME	FOOD	AMOUNT	CALORIES

TRIGGER TRACKER

IMMEDIATELY AFTER	AFTER 1 HOUR	AFTER 3 HOUR

Date _____

	LOW	MED	HIGH
SLEEP QUALITY	○	○	○
ENERGY LEVEL	○	○	○
ACTIVITY LEVEL	○	○	○

MY MOOD

- Relaxed
- Happy
- Inspired
- Angry
- Tired
- Stressed
- _____

TODAY'S GOALS

- _____
- _____
- _____

MEDICATIONS

- _____
- _____
- _____

SUPPLEMENTS

- _____
- _____
- _____

CURRENT WEIGHT

WATER INTAKE

NOTES

_____
_____
_____
_____
_____
_____

FOOD LOG

TIME	FOOD	AMOUNT	CALORIES

TRIGGER TRACKER

IMMEDIATELY AFTER	AFTER 1 HOUR	AFTER 3 HOUR

Date _____

	LOW	MED	HIGH
SLEEP QUALITY	●	●	●
ENERGY LEVEL	●	●	●
ACTIVITY LEVEL	●	●	●

MY MOOD

- ● Relaxed
- ● Happy
- ● Inspired
- ● Angry
- ● Tired
- ● Stressed
- ● _____

TODAY'S GOALS

- ● _____
- ● _____
- ● _____

MEDICATIONS

- ● _____
- ● _____
- ● _____

CURRENT WEIGHT

SUPPLEMENTS

- ● _____
- ● _____
- ● _____

WATER INTAKE

NOTES

_____
_____
_____
_____
_____
_____

FOOD LOG

TIME	FOOD	AMOUNT	CALORIES

TRIGGER TRACKER

IMMEDIATELY AFTER	AFTER 1 HOUR	AFTER 3 HOUR

Date _____

	LOW	MED	HIGH
SLEEP QUALITY	◯	◯	◯
ENERGY LEVEL	◯	◯	◯
ACTIVITY LEVEL	◯	◯	◯

MY MOOD

- Relaxed
- Happy
- Inspired
- Angry
- Tired
- Stressed
- _____

TODAY'S GOALS

- _____
- _____
- _____

MEDICATIONS

- _____
- _____
- _____

CURRENT WEIGHT

SUPPLEMENTS

- _____
- _____
- _____

WATER INTAKE

💧 💧 💧 💧 💧
💧 💧 💧 💧 💧
💧 💧 💧 💧 💧

NOTES

_____
_____
_____
_____
_____
_____

FOOD LOG

TIME	FOOD	AMOUNT	CALORIES

TRIGGER TRACKER

IMMEDIATELY AFTER	AFTER 1 HOUR	AFTER 3 HOUR

Date _____

SLEEP QUALITY
ENERGY LEVEL
ACTIVITY LEVEL

LOW   MED   HIGH

MY MOOD

- Relaxed
- Happy
- Inspired
- Angry
- Tired
- Stressed
- _____

TODAY'S GOALS

- _____
- _____
- _____

MEDICATIONS

- _____
- _____
- _____

CURRENT WEIGHT

SUPPLEMENTS

- _____
- _____
- _____

WATER INTAKE

NOTES

_____
_____
_____
_____
_____
_____

FOOD LOG

TIME	FOOD	AMOUNT	CALORIES

TRIGGER TRACKER

IMMEDIATELY AFTER	AFTER 1 HOUR	AFTER 3 HOUR

Date _____

MY MOOD

- Relaxed
- Happy
- Inspired
- Angry
- Tired
- Stressed
- _____

	LOW	MED	HIGH
SLEEP QUALITY	●	●	●
ENERGY LEVEL	●	●	●
ACTIVITY LEVEL	●	●	●

TODAY'S GOALS

- _____
- _____
- _____

MEDICATIONS

- _____
- _____
- _____

CURRENT WEIGHT

SUPPLEMENTS

- _____
- _____
- _____

WATER INTAKE

NOTES

_____
_____
_____
_____
_____
_____

FOOD LOG

TIME	FOOD	AMOUNT	CALORIES

TRIGGER TRACKER

IMMEDIATELY AFTER	AFTER 1 HOUR	AFTER 3 HOUR

Date _____

	LOW	MED	HIGH
SLEEP QUALITY	○	○	○
ENERGY LEVEL	○	○	○
ACTIVITY LEVEL	○	○	○

MY MOOD

- Relaxed
- Happy
- Inspired
- Angry
- Tired
- Stressed
- _____

TODAY'S GOALS

- _____
- _____
- _____

MEDICATIONS

- _____
- _____
- _____

CURRENT WEIGHT

SUPPLEMENTS

- _____
- _____
- _____

WATER INTAKE

NOTES

_____
_____
_____
_____
_____
_____

FOOD LOG

TIME	FOOD	AMOUNT	CALORIES

TRIGGER TRACKER

IMMEDIATELY AFTER	AFTER 1 HOUR	AFTER 3 HOUR

Date _____

	LOW	MED	HIGH
SLEEP QUALITY	○	○	●
ENERGY LEVEL	○	○	●
ACTIVITY LEVEL	○	○	●

MY MOOD

- ○ Relaxed
- ○ Happy
- ○ Inspired
- ○ Angry
- ○ Tired
- ○ Stressed
- ○ _____

TODAY'S GOALS

- ○ _____
- ○ _____
- ○ _____

MEDICATIONS

- ○ _____
- ○ _____
- ○ _____

SUPPLEMENTS

- ○ _____
- ○ _____
- ○ _____

CURRENT WEIGHT

WATER INTAKE

💧 💧 💧 💧 💧
💧 💧 💧 💧 💧
💧 💧 💧 💧 💧

NOTES

_____
_____
_____
_____
_____
_____

FOOD LOG

TIME	FOOD	AMOUNT	CALORIES

TRIGGER TRACKER

IMMEDIATELY AFTER	AFTER 1 HOUR	AFTER 3 HOUR

Date _____

MY MOOD

- Relaxed
- Happy
- Inspired
- Angry
- Tired
- Stressed
- _____

	LOW	MED	HIGH
SLEEP QUALITY	●	●	●
ENERGY LEVEL	●	●	●
ACTIVITY LEVEL	●	●	●

TODAY'S GOALS

- _____
- _____
- _____

MEDICATIONS

- _____
- _____
- _____

CURRENT WEIGHT

WATER INTAKE

SUPPLEMENTS

- _____
- _____
- _____

NOTES

_____
_____
_____
_____
_____
_____

FOOD LOG

TIME	FOOD	AMOUNT	CALORIES

TRIGGER TRACKER

IMMEDIATELY AFTER	AFTER 1 HOUR	AFTER 3 HOUR

Date _____

MY MOOD

	LOW	MED	HIGH
SLEEP QUALITY	●	●	●
ENERGY LEVEL	●	●	●
ACTIVITY LEVEL	●	●	●

● Relaxed
● Happy
● Inspired
● Angry
● Tired
● Stressed
● _____

TODAY'S GOALS

● _____
● _____
● _____

MEDICATIONS

● _____
● _____
● _____

CURRENT WEIGHT

SUPPLEMENTS

● _____
● _____
● _____

WATER INTAKE

NOTES

_____
_____
_____
_____
_____
_____

FOOD LOG

TIME	FOOD	AMOUNT	CALORIES

TRIGGER TRACKER

IMMEDIATELY AFTER	AFTER 1 HOUR	AFTER 3 HOUR

Date _____

MY MOOD

- ⬤ Relaxed
- ⬤ Happy
- ⬤ Inspired
- ⬤ Angry
- ⬤ Tired
- ⬤ Stressed
- ⬤ _____

	LOW	MED	HIGH
SLEEP QUALITY	⬤	⬤	⬤
ENERGY LEVEL	⬤	⬤	⬤
ACTIVITY LEVEL	⬤	⬤	⬤

TODAY'S GOALS

- ⬤ _____
- ⬤ _____
- ⬤ _____

MEDICATIONS

- ⬤ _____
- ⬤ _____
- ⬤ _____

CURRENT WEIGHT

WATER INTAKE

SUPPLEMENTS

- ⬤ _____
- ⬤ _____
- ⬤ _____

NOTES

_____
_____
_____
_____
_____
_____

FOOD LOG

TIME	FOOD	AMOUNT	CALORIES

TRIGGER TRACKER

IMMEDIATELY AFTER	AFTER 1 HOUR	AFTER 3 HOUR

Date _____

MY MOOD

SLEEP QUALITY   LOW   MED   HIGH

ENERGY LEVEL

ACTIVITY LEVEL

- Relaxed
- Happy
- Inspired
- Angry
- Tired
- Stressed
- _____

TODAY'S GOALS

- _____
- _____
- _____

MEDICATIONS

- _____
- _____
- _____

CURRENT WEIGHT

WATER INTAKE

SUPPLEMENTS

- _____
- _____
- _____

NOTES

_____
_____
_____
_____
_____
_____

FOOD LOG

TIME	FOOD	AMOUNT	CALORIES

TRIGGER TRACKER

IMMEDIATELY AFTER	AFTER 1 HOUR	AFTER 3 HOUR

Date _____

MY MOOD

SLEEP QUALITY   LOW   MED   HIGH

ENERGY LEVEL

ACTIVITY LEVEL

- Relaxed
- Happy
- Inspired
- Angry
- Tired
- Stressed
- _____

TODAY'S GOALS

- _____
- _____
- _____

MEDICATIONS

- _____
- _____
- _____

CURRENT WEIGHT

WATER INTAKE

SUPPLEMENTS

- _____
- _____
- _____

NOTES

_____
_____
_____
_____
_____
_____

FOOD LOG

TIME	FOOD	AMOUNT	CALORIES

TRIGGER TRACKER

IMMEDIATELY AFTER	AFTER 1 HOUR	AFTER 3 HOUR

Date _____

	LOW	MED	HIGH
SLEEP QUALITY	○	○	○
ENERGY LEVEL	○	○	○
ACTIVITY LEVEL	○	○	○

MY MOOD

- ● Relaxed
- ● Happy
- ● Inspired
- ● Angry
- ● Tired
- ● Stressed
- ● _____

TODAY'S GOALS

- ● _____
- ● _____
- ● _____

MEDICATIONS

- ● _____
- ● _____
- ● _____

CURRENT WEIGHT

WATER INTAKE

SUPPLEMENTS

- ● _____
- ● _____
- ● _____

NOTES

_____
_____
_____
_____
_____
_____

FOOD LOG

TIME	FOOD	AMOUNT	CALORIES

TRIGGER TRACKER

IMMEDIATELY AFTER	AFTER 1 HOUR	AFTER 3 HOUR

Date _____

	LOW	MED	HIGH
SLEEP QUALITY	○	○	○
ENERGY LEVEL	○	○	○
ACTIVITY LEVEL	○	○	○

MY MOOD

○ Relaxed
○ Happy
○ Inspired
○ Angry
○ Tired
○ Stressed
○ _____

TODAY'S GOALS

○ _____
○ _____
○ _____

MEDICATIONS

○ _____
○ _____
○ _____

CURRENT WEIGHT

WATER INTAKE

SUPPLEMENTS

○ _____
○ _____
○ _____

NOTES

_____
_____
_____
_____
_____
_____
_____

FOOD LOG

TIME	FOOD	AMOUNT	CALORIES

TRIGGER TRACKER

IMMEDIATELY AFTER	AFTER 1 HOUR	AFTER 3 HOUR

Date _____

MY MOOD

SLEEP QUALITY — LOW MED HIGH

ENERGY LEVEL

ACTIVITY LEVEL

- Relaxed
- Happy
- Inspired
- Angry
- Tired
- Stressed
- _____

TODAY'S GOALS

- _____
- _____
- _____

MEDICATIONS

- _____
- _____
- _____

CURRENT WEIGHT

WATER INTAKE

SUPPLEMENTS

- _____
- _____
- _____

NOTES

_____
_____
_____
_____
_____
_____

FOOD LOG

TIME	FOOD	AMOUNT	CALORIES

TRIGGER TRACKER

IMMEDIATELY AFTER	AFTER 1 HOUR	AFTER 3 HOUR

Date _____

MY MOOD

- Relaxed
- Happy
- Inspired
- Angry
- Tired
- Stressed
- _____

	LOW	MED	HIGH
SLEEP QUALITY	○	○	○
ENERGY LEVEL	○	○	○
ACTIVITY LEVEL	○	○	○

TODAY'S GOALS

- _____
- _____
- _____

MEDICATIONS

- _____
- _____
- _____

CURRENT WEIGHT

WATER INTAKE

SUPPLEMENTS

- _____
- _____
- _____

NOTES

_____
_____
_____
_____
_____
_____
_____

FOOD LOG

TIME	FOOD	AMOUNT	CALORIES

TRIGGER TRACKER

IMMEDIATELY AFTER	AFTER 1 HOUR	AFTER 3 HOUR

Date _____

	LOW	MED	HIGH
SLEEP QUALITY	○	○	○
ENERGY LEVEL	○	○	○
ACTIVITY LEVEL	○	○	○

MY MOOD

- Relaxed
- Happy
- Inspired
- Angry
- Tired
- Stressed
- _____

TODAY'S GOALS

- _____
- _____
- _____

MEDICATIONS

- _____
- _____
- _____

CURRENT WEIGHT

SUPPLEMENTS

- _____
- _____
- _____

WATER INTAKE

NOTES

_____
_____
_____
_____
_____
_____

FOOD LOG

TIME	FOOD	AMOUNT	CALORIES

TRIGGER TRACKER

IMMEDIATELY AFTER	AFTER 1 HOUR	AFTER 3 HOUR

Date _____

MY MOOD

- Relaxed
- Happy
- Inspired
- Angry
- Tired
- Stressed
- _____

	LOW	MED	HIGH
SLEEP QUALITY	●	●	●
ENERGY LEVEL	●	●	●
ACTIVITY LEVEL	●	●	●

TODAY'S GOALS

- _____
- _____
- _____

MEDICATIONS

- _____
- _____
- _____

CURRENT WEIGHT

SUPPLEMENTS

- _____
- _____
- _____

WATER INTAKE

NOTES

_____
_____
_____
_____
_____

FOOD LOG

TIME	FOOD	AMOUNT	CALORIES

TRIGGER TRACKER

IMMEDIATELY AFTER	AFTER 1 HOUR	AFTER 3 HOUR

Made in the USA
Middletown, DE
23 November 2024

65267418R00070